The Anti Aging Secret of the Animals – Learn the Simple Somatic Movements That Can Cure Back Pain, Restore Your Flexibility and Rejuvenate Your Body to Its Natural, Youthful State Today!

By Anthony Anholt

Copyright © 2013 by Anthony Anholt

Discover other fitness titles by Anthony Anholt on Kindle:

The Isometric Exercise Bible

The Bodyweight Exercise Bible

The Abdominal Exercise Bible

Jump Rope Workouts

Tapping Scripts for Beginners

The Breathing Exercise Bible

Disclaimer

The exercises and advice contained within this course may be too strenuous or dangerous for some people, and the reader(s) should consult a physician before engaging in them. The author and publisher of this course are not responsible in any manner whatsoever for any injury which may occur through reading and following the instructions herein.

Table of Contents

Why Do Our Bodies Wear Down?

How old would you be if you didn't know how old you are? – Satchel Paige

Do you remember how great your body felt when you were young? Flexible and strong, it could do anything and take you anywhere with little effort. When you were a teenager you likely bounded out of bed in the morning without giving it a second thought. Anything you wanted to do you could do. Run, jump, play any sport you wanted. Wasn't it great?

As we begin to age, however, things begin to change. For most of us as early as our mid twenties we start to acquire little aches and pains that make us realize that we're not as young as we used to be. Whereas before we would seemingly instantly recover from any athletic activity it now wears on us. What's worse is that overtime these little aches and pains start to accumulate. People react to this new reality in various ways. Some people try and fight it with a combination of drugs like Ibuprofen and shear stubbornness. Others, unfortunately, give up and simply cut back on or even eliminate the activities and sports they once enjoyed. As the years fly by many people's bodies seem to degenerate to the point where even the most basic movements become difficult. Getting out of bed can become a struggle and walking requires a cane. Most people simply accept this as being a part of the natural aging process. It's simply a fact of life and nothing can be done about it. Right? Wrong!

The fact of the matter is that it is not true that aging and increasing decrepitude walk hand in hand. Consider our animal friends in nature. Do their bodies start to fall apart as they age? Have you ever seen a Cheetah running at full speed having to stop due to a pulled hamstring? Why is it that the aging process is seemingly so different between our animal relatives and us? Can we learn something from them?

The answer, it won't surprise you, is yes. The fact of the matter is that all vertebrate mammals posses incredible self-healing abilities. By instinct all mammals are able to access these abilities to keep their bodies in tiptop shape, including humans. The problem for human beings is that as our higher brain functions become active we lose these instincts. This book is all about teaching you to regain this animal anti-aging instinct so that you can rejuvenate your body and feel great again, no matter what your age.

Understanding The Brains Role

Modern medicine, for all its advances, knows less than 10 percent of what your body knows instinctively – Deepak Chopra

The human brain is similar to an immensely powerful computer that controls our thoughts, movements, memories and decisions. An evolutionary marvel, it is made up of billions of brain cells that send and receive information at the speed of light. The structures that make up the oldest parts of the human brain are largely shared and indistinguishable from our animal (mammal) friends. What makes the human brain unique however is its immense size. In fact our brains are three times larger than the brains of similar sized mammals. The reason for this is the cerebral cortex (otherwise known as the cortical part of the brain) which is extremely developed in humans and therefore quite large. Located on the outside of the brain the cortex grants us the ability to mull over the past, prepare for the future, and analyze abstract situations and problems. This part of the brain is what really makes us human and gives us the brainpower to create everything from striped toothpaste to airplanes. In life, however, it is often the case that for every positive, no matter how great, there is often a negative and it is true in this case as well. Although our reliance on our cerebral cortex brings many benefits it also limits us in that it can overwhelm our more basic instincts from our more ancient subcortical brain. This is why so many of suffer from increased aches and pains as we age.

To better understand this concept it is helpful to look at the brain as a computer. The cerebral cortex, or cortical parts of the brain, is like the RAM in a computer in that it readily accepts new instructions to be carried out. When you are learning something new for the first time, such as swinging a tennis racquet, this is the part of the brain you are using.

The subcortical part of the brain is like the firmware or ROM parts of a computer. Instructions are much more permanent here and are much harder to change. Bodily functions such as keeping your heart beating and regulating your breath are controlled here. Automatic reactions such as instantly pulling your hand back if you touch a hot stove are rooted in your subcortical brain. When you accidently touch a hot object you don't have to think about it. Instead, your subcortical brain takes over in order to save you from danger. These kinds of instructions were likely programmed into our brain during caveman times and they haven't changed much since then.

How does this knowledge of the cortical and subcortical parts of the brain relate to rejuvenating your body? Here's how. As you live your life you will experience both mental and physical trauma. For example most of us have had the experience where we have attempted to lift a heavy object only to feel anything from a twinge to an intense pain from our back. This is obviously an example of physical trauma. What is going on here is that our conscious, cortical part of our brain is attempting to carry out an instruction to lift a heavy object. However the object you are lifting is too heavy and the possibility exists that you might injure yourself. This is where the subcortical brain takes over in order to protect you. Without you having to think about it your back muscles spasm or seize up and you drop the heavy object. This kind of reaction is exactly the same kind of response you get if you were to touch that hot stove. Without thinking your subcortical brain instantly reacts to protect you from harm.

Although it is typically a slower process emotional trauma can have the same physical effect on your body. For example, let's say you are facing a tight deadline at work that you are worried you might miss. Although the trauma you are experiencing is purely mental your sub cortex will attempt to protect you in a physical way. This is why various muscles will tense up and you are much more vulnerable to conditions like back spasms when you are stressed. Once again your subcortical brain is simply trying to protect you.

The problem with the above is that once the trauma has passed our subcortical brain sometimes doesn't completely release the muscles it has tightened. You can feel the muscles that are tight because they are likely sore but you can't find a way to relax them. Thomas Hanna, author of "Somatics", calls this "sensory motor amnesia". The firmware or ROM in your subcortical brain has become corrupted and will not allow the muscles to relax. With your subcortical brain in charge your cerebral cortex looses the ability to relax the previously traumatized muscles. What is worse is that these same tight muscles cause your body to become out of alignment. The brain attempts to compensate for this by using other muscles, which can then cause further trauma. It can be a slow process, but overtime these conditions compound on each other until we are simply sore all the time. Most people interpret this reality as the price of "getting older", but it doesn't have to be this way. In order to really solve this issue what is needed is a way to "reset" the faulty instructions that our subcortical brain has acquired. Going back to my computer analogy it is sometimes necessary to "clear out the cache" in order for the computer to perform well. This is the same idea, except we want to reset our brains. When we are able to program our sub cortical brain to release the muscles under its control they will relax and we will no longer be exerting the energy keeping those muscles tight. This is the key to returning your body to a dynamic youthful state and thankfully it is an ability that all vertebrate mammals have, including you.

What Is The Animals Secret?

Too many people, when they get old, think that they have to live by the calendar – John Glenn

If you are like most people you likely feel a little stiff when you first wake up in the morning. Ever wonder why this is? The reason is that our muscles are designed to do one thing and one thing only and that is to contract. When we move throughout the day our muscles are continually contracting and releasing which is why they stay at least somewhat loose. However, when we sleep we don't move that much and our muscles only contract, hence the stiffness. This is true of all vertebrate animals, not just human beings. This is why all animals appear to stretch when they first wake up. If you have a cat or dog you have likely observed this first hand. What will likely surprise you though is that these animals are not stretching at all in the way that we understand it, they are pandiculating. This is the anti-aging secret of the animals and it is what this little book is going to show you how to do too.

Take a look at the picture of the big cat below. You might think it is stretching (often call a cat stretch) but it isn't. What it is really doing is contracting its back muscles in order to form an arch. Any "stretch" it gets along its stomach is completely incidental. When it releases this forced contraction the back muscles loosen and become limber. The brain also releases powerful chemicals to relax the muscles that have just contracted. This process is called pandiculation. During a pandiculation the muscles are contracted and then relaxed, which allows the brain to reset them.

Human beings, when they are in the womb and are first born, perform these kinds of movements as well by instinct. As our higher brain functions become active however it is an instinct we lose. That's the bad news. The good news is that by conscious movement we can learn to pandiculate and regain control of our muscles and brain once again.

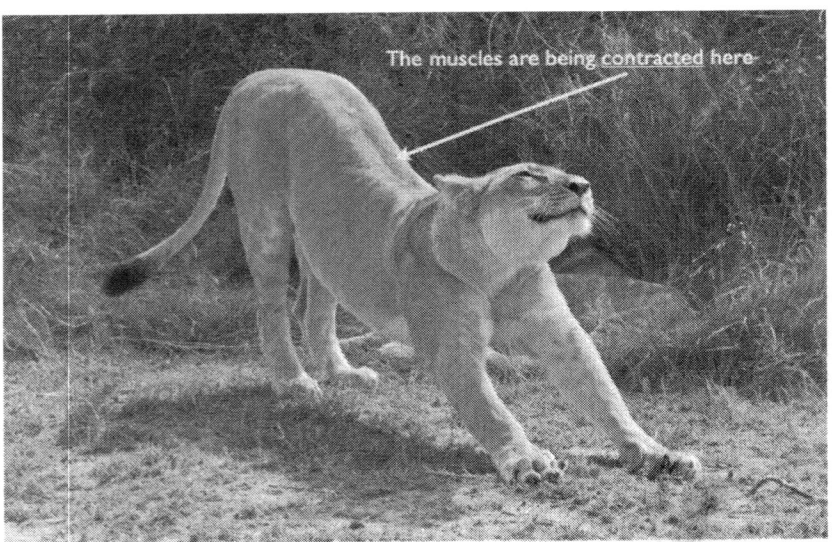

The muscles are being contracted here

This lion is not stretching, it is pandiculating. This is the key to how all vertebrate mammals maintain their youthful flexibility.

Restoring Youthful Flexibility

Grow old along with me! The best is yet to be
– Robert Browning

So now that we understand how other mammals retain their youthful flexibility throughout their lives how can we make use of it? The key is to perform simple movements slowly with conscious intention. Done properly this allows us to reset or reboot our subcortical brain, allowing our cerebral cortex to regain control and relax those muscles. This is sometimes known as somatic exercise which is a term coined by Thomas Hanna who largely developed the technique. From my experience I hesitate to call them exercises as this invokes thoughts in people of hard work. Exercise means sweating and working your muscles, which is the exact opposite of what we are trying to do. Rather than working your muscles we are attempting to work your mind so that we can reset it. This is why from now on I will only refer to somatic movements rather than somatic exercises.

The somatic movements you are about to perform all fit within a five-point pattern that you will perform each time. They are:

Prepare – Get you body in the required position so that you can perform the somatic movement. It is always a good idea to close your eyes and keep them closed throughout the movement so that you can concentrate on how the muscles are feeling.

Move Slowly – Gently and slowly perform the somatic movement. Always keep your mind focused internally on how your muscles are feeling.

Release Slowly – Typically means to reverse the movement you have just performed.

Relax – Perhaps the most import part of the movement. Simply take a deep breath through your nose and relax. If you felt any tightness in your muscles focus your mind on relaxing them.

Repeat – For most of these somatic movements I provide you with a minimum number that you should perform. However, always remember these are only guidelines. If you sense that your body needs more feel free to do more. These are not exercises so you cannot tire yourself out. Do as many as you feel are helpful.

Following this five point protocol will allow your cortical brain to re-assert control over your subcortical brain. It is deceptively easy to do but therein lays the potential danger. If you do not perform these movements slowly and with intention you run the risk of using your subcortical brain, which will completely defeat the purpose. Always remember that when your brain is focused and paying attention you are using your cortical brain. When you are doing things on automatic pilot you are likely using your subcortical brain. The former is desirable while the latter is not.

What's Next?

What follows are some rules that I always want you to keep in mind when performing your somatic movements. From there we will get into the movements themselves. For the first week I want you to focus on a single somatic movement. The goal here is to get used to the gentle movement and working your mind and body from within. From there I will offer you two short somatic sequences from which you will choose one, depending on your circumstances. Finally I will show you the "cat stretch", which is a series of somatic movements you can perform everyday if you wish.

Somatic Movement Rules

Always move with intention and awareness

When performing any of the following somatic movements always keep the following rules in mind.

Rule 1 - Always remember that somatic exercises are not traditional exercises designed to work your muscles – they are brain-reset movements.

You should only be moving your limbs though space and concentrating on the feeling this generates inside your body. At no time should you be sweating or straining.

Rule 2 – Always perform these somatic movements slowly and with focused attention.

If you perform these movements too quickly you run the risk of using your sub-cortical brain which will prevent it from being re-programmed. Going slowly and focusing on how you feel allows your cortical brain to take the lead and re-assert control over your muscles.

Rule 3 – Never perform these movements to the point of discomfort or strain. Always stay well within your comfort zone.

Again, these are not exercises. At the slightest hint of discomfort you need to back off.

Rule 4 – Always remember that the provided pictures are for guidance only.

Do not be concerned in the least if you cannot match the pictures provided for the movement. Only do what you can do. Always concentrate on how your muscles feel, not on how you look doing a movement. It is fine if you only feel comfortable moving a fraction of an inch.

Rule 5 – Always perform these movements with your eyes closed.

Your goal at all times is to focus your mind internally with regards to how your muscles are feeling. Closed eyes aide greatly in this whereas open ones lead to distractions.

Your First Somatic Movement

What follows here is a simple somatic movement that is excellent for your lower back. Even if you are one of the lucky few that does not have any kind of lower back pain I suggest you do it anyway so that you get a feel for what somatic movement is all about. Perform this movement for a couple of days until you feel comfortable with it before moving onto somatic sequences A and B. Of course you can do this movement anytime you want as well. First thing in the morning works well for most people.

Somatic Movement #1 – For Lower Back Pain

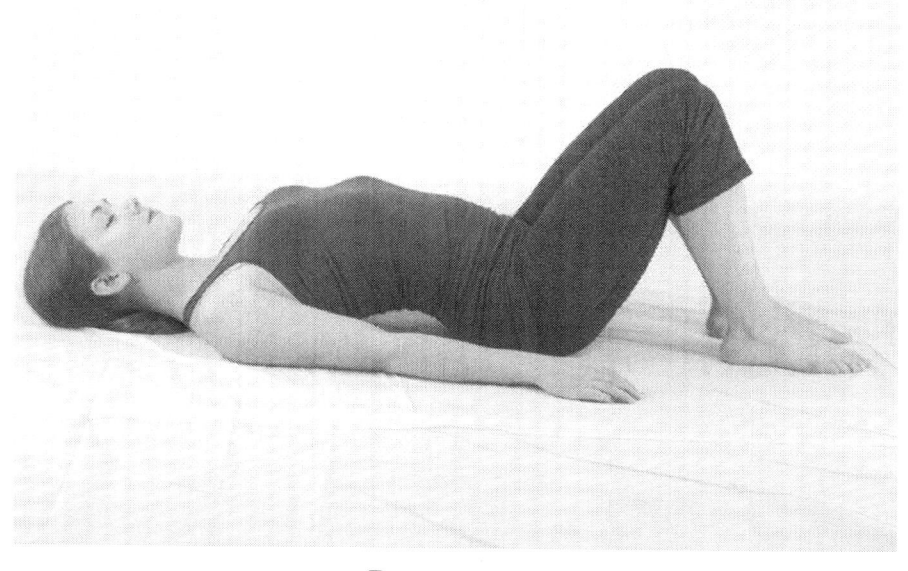

Prepare

Begin by lying flat on your back with your knees bent and your eyes closed.

Move Slowly

Inhale through your nose as you gently press your tailbone downwards. This will cause your lower back to arch up. Move slowly and focus on the sensations this movement causes within your body.

Release Slowly

Slowly exhale through your mouth as you gently thrust your pelvis slightly upward, which will flatten the arch in your back. Again focus on how your muscles feel as you do this. Take special note of any muscles that seem to feel extra tense.

Relax

Slowly inhale through your nose and exhale through your mouth. As you do so focus your mind on the sensations you have just felt. If you felt any tension in your body focus your mind on relaxing those muscles or areas.

Repeat

Do this movement for a minimum of 5 times. Do more if you sense that your body needs it.

Somatic Sequence A

This simple somatic sequence is ideal for people who tend to lean forward when they walk or stand. It can also help those who are prone to back spasms. If this sounds like you give it a try for a week before moving onto the cat stretch. Of course there is the possibility that this sequence is all you need in which case feel free to do it as long as you want. It's all up to you and what your body needs and feels.

Holistic Movement #1 – Somatic Sequence A

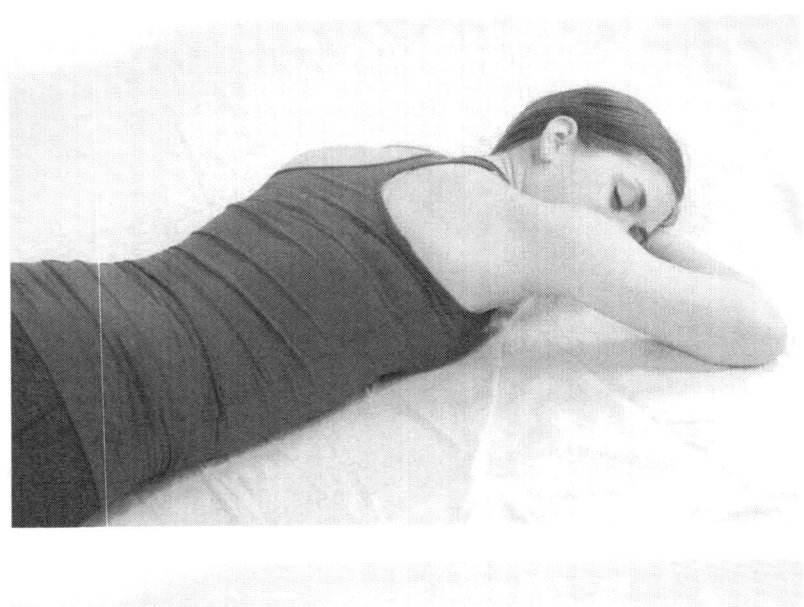

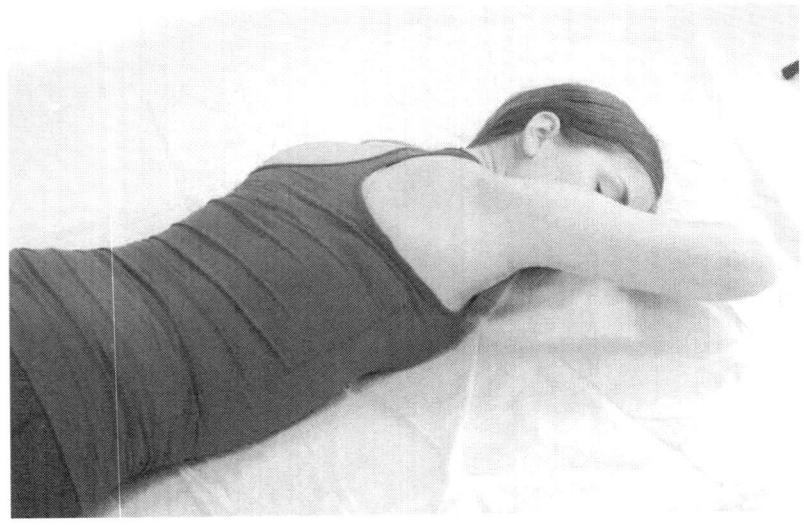

Holistic Movement #1 – Somatic Sequence A

Prepare

Begin by lying flat on your stomach. Turn your head to the right and place your right hand under your left cheek. Your left arm should remain resting alongside your body. Close your eyes and keep them closed.

Move Slowly

Inhale through your nose as you gently lift up your right elbow. Which muscles feel tight to you?

Release Slowly

Slowly exhale through your mouth as you lower your right elbow back to the floor.

Relax

Slowly inhale through your nose and exhale through your mouth. As you do so focus your mind on the sensations you have just felt. If you felt any tension in your body focus your mind on relaxing those muscles or areas of your body.

Repeat

Do this movement for a minimum of 3 times. Then repeat this movement using the opposite side of your body (by placing your left hand under your right cheek).

Holistic Movement #2 – Somatic Sequence A

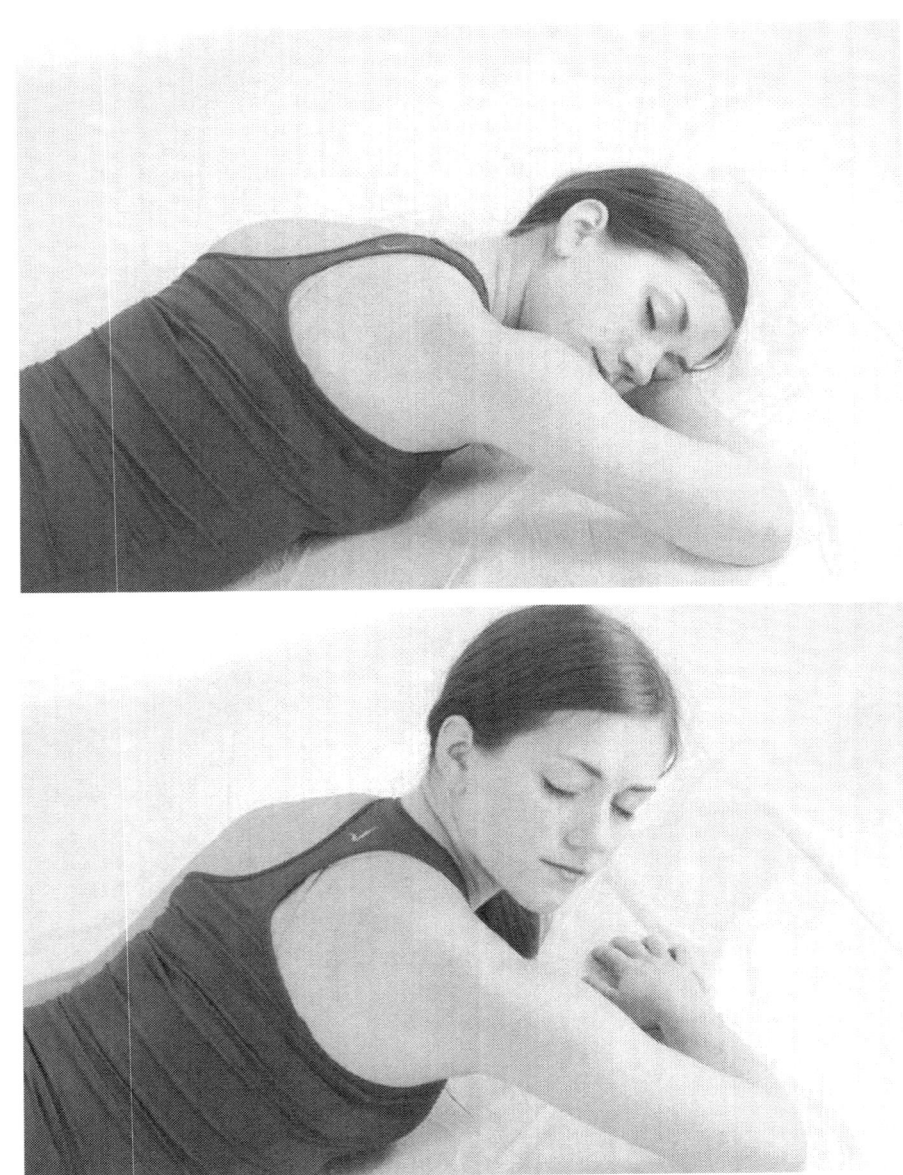

Holistic Movement #2 – Somatic Sequence A

Prepare

Begin by lying flat on your stomach. Turn your head to the right and place your right hand under your left cheek. Your left arm should remain resting alongside your body with your eyes closed.

Move Slowly

Inhale through your nose as you slowly lift your head (not your arm) in order to look over your right shoulder. Make sure you are well within your comfort zone when you do this, you should not feel any strain at all. Take note of where the muscles are contracting.

Release Slowly

Slowly exhale through your mouth as you lower your head back to the ground.

Relax

Slowly inhale through your nose and exhale through your mouth. As you do so focus your mind on the sensations you have just felt. If you felt any tension in your body focus your mind on relaxing those muscles or areas of your body.

Repeat

Do this movement for a minimum of 3 times. Then repeat this movement using the opposite side of your body (by looking over your left shoulder 3 times).

Holistic Movement #3 – Somatic Sequence A

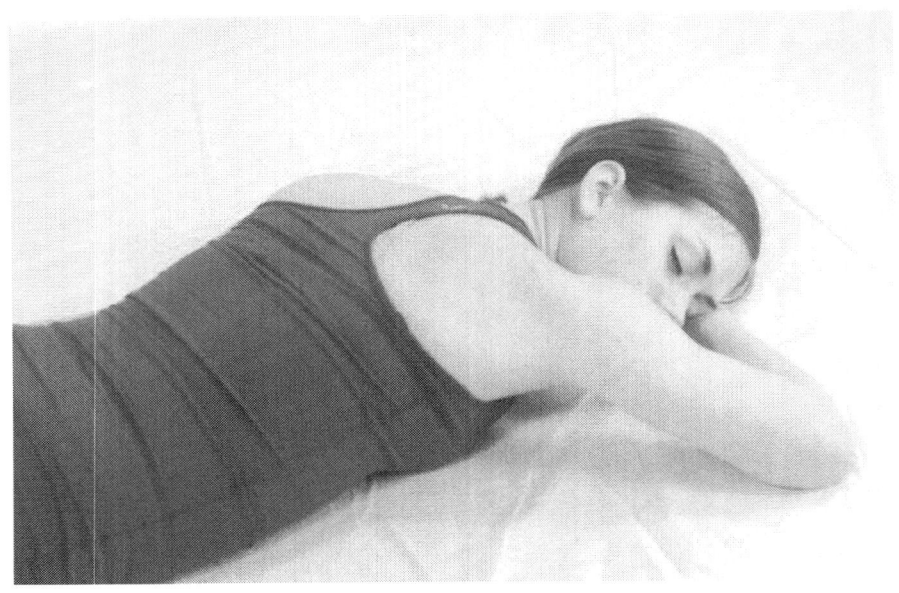

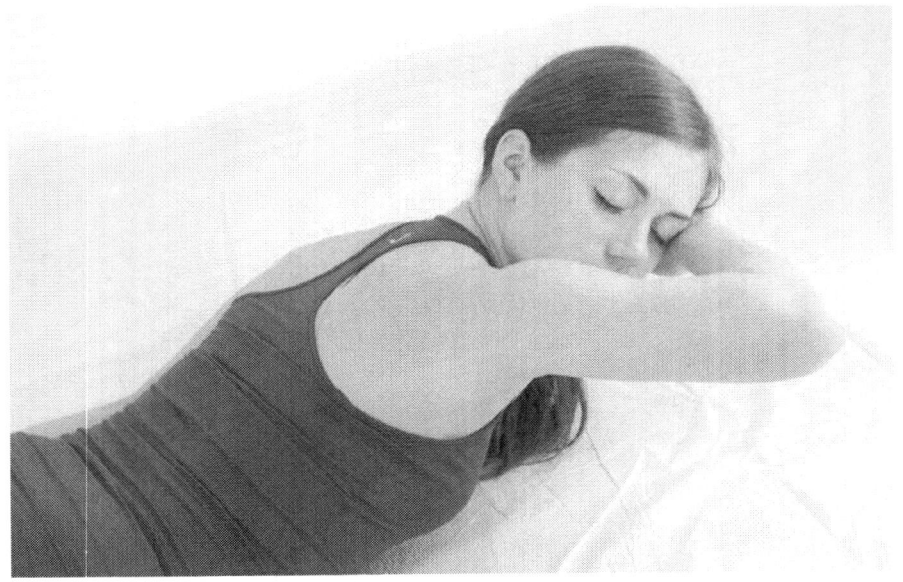

Holistic Movement #3 – Somatic Sequence A

Prepare

Begin by lying flat on your stomach. Turn your head to the right and place your right hand under your left cheek. Your left arm should remain resting alongside your body. Close your eyes and keep them closed throughout the movement.

Move Slowly

Inhale through your nose as you look over your right shoulder by lifting your elbow, hand and head at the same time. Which muscles are contracting now? How does this feel different from the first 2 variations?

Release Slowly

Slowly exhale through your mouth as you lower your head and arm back to the ground.

Relax

Slowly inhale through your nose and exhale through your mouth. As you do so focus your mind on the sensations you have just felt. If you felt any tension in your body focus your mind on relaxing those muscles or areas of your body.

Repeat

Do this movement for a minimum of 3 times. Then repeat this movement using the opposite side of your body (by looking over your left shoulder 3 times).

Holistic Movement #4 – Somatic Sequence A

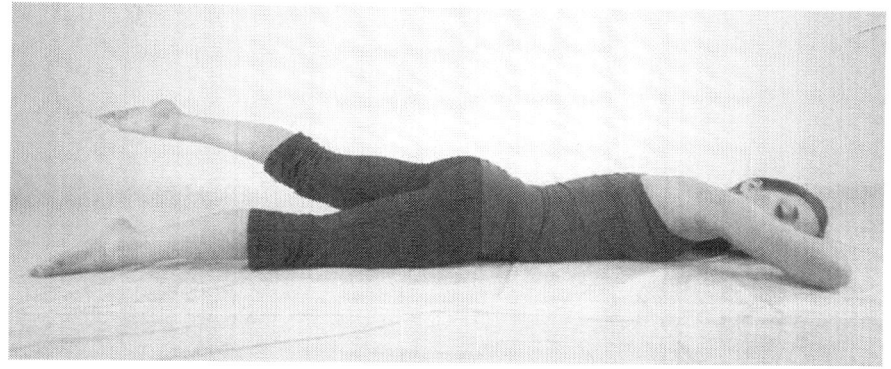

Prepare

Begin by lying flat on your stomach. Turn your head to the right and place your right hand under your left cheek. Your left arm should remain resting alongside your body with your eyes closed.

Move Slowly

Inhale through your nose as you slowly and gently lift your left leg a few inches off the floor. Once again do not strain yourself. Always remember this is a movement, not an exercise. You shouldn't strain your muscles at all.

Release Slowly

Slowly exhale through your mouth as you lower your leg back to the ground.

Relax

Slowly inhale through your nose and exhale through your mouth. As you do so focus your mind on the sensations you have just felt. Did you feel any tension in your spine or shoulder? Focus your mind on relaxing those muscles or any area of your body where you felt tension.

Repeat

Do this movement for a minimum of 3 times. Then repeat this movement by reversing it (turning your head to the left and lifting your right leg).

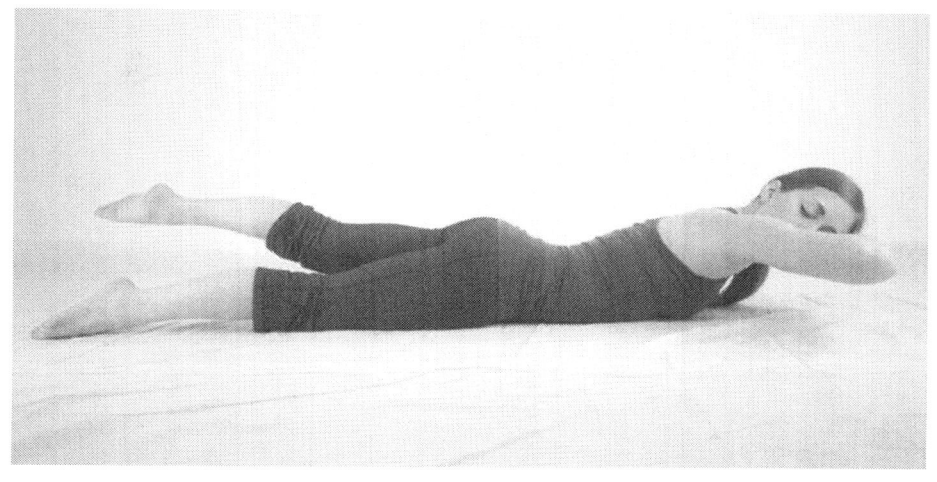

Prepare

Begin by lying flat on your stomach. Turn your head to the right and place your right hand under your left cheek. Your left arm should remain beside your body. Close your eyes and keep them closed throughout the movement.

Move Slowly

Inhale through your nose as you slowly and gently lift your left leg a few inches off the floor along with your head, hand and elbow. You should feel no strain when doing this.

Release Slowly

Slowly exhale through your mouth as you lower your leg and head back to the ground.

Relax

Slowly inhale through your nose and exhale through your mouth. Focus your mind on removing any tension you may have felt.

Repeat

Do this movement for a minimum of 3 times. Then repeat this movement by reversing it (turning your head to the left and lifting your head and right leg).

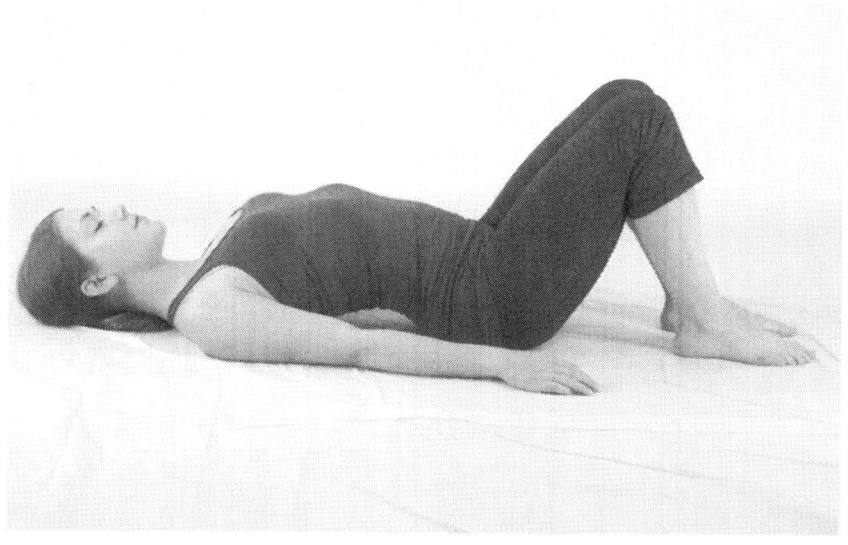

Prepare

In order to balance things out we will now repeat the first somatic movement you learned. Once again begin by lying flat on your back with your knees bent. As a variation though try starting with your feet closer together or further apart and see how this feels. Close your eyes.

Move Slowly

Inhale through your nose as you gently press your tailbone downwards. This will cause your lower back to arch up. Move slowly and focus on the sensations this movement causes within your body.

Release Slowly

Slowly exhale through your mouth as you gently thrust your pelvis slightly upward, which will flatten the arch in your back and press it to the floor. Again focus on how your muscles feel as you do this. Take special note of any that seem to feel extra tense.

Relax

Slowly inhale through your nose and exhale through your mouth. As you do so focus your mind on the sensations you have just felt. If you felt any tension in your body focus your mind on relaxing those muscles or areas of your body .

Repeat

Do this movement for a minimum of 5 times. Do more if you sense that your body needs it.

Somatic Sequence B

This simple somatic sequence is ideal for people who spend a great part of their day sitting. The truth of the matter is that sitting in a chair or in a car for extended periods is one of the worst things you can do for your back. If you spend a great deal of time sitting try this somatic sequence for a week. You may find this routine is all you need to feel great again.

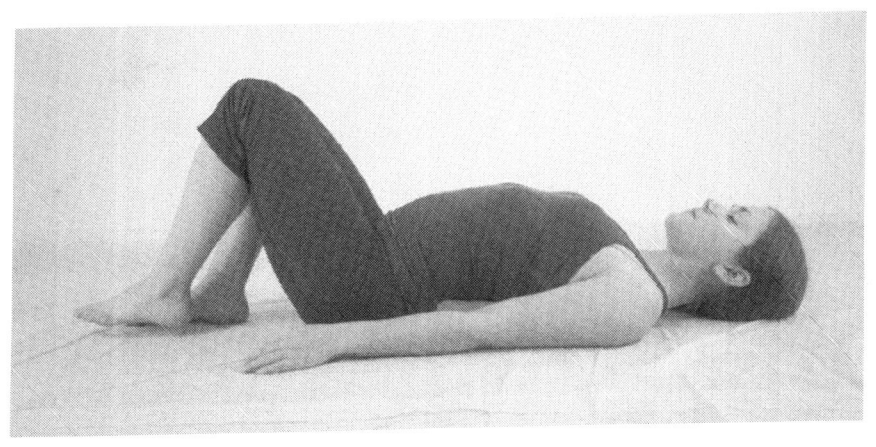

Prepare

Begin by lying flat on your back with your knees bent and eyes closed.

Move Slowly

Inhale through your nose as you gently and slowly press your tailbone downwards while simultaneously lifting your left foot off the ground. You should endeavor to lift your foot as little as possible. Take note of whatever sensations you feel in your muscles.

Release Slowly

Slowly exhale through your mouth as you gently relax your tailbone and lower your foot back to the ground.

Relax

Slowly inhale through your nose and exhale through your mouth. Focus your mind on whatever tension your feel and command those muscles to relax.

Repeat

Do this movement for a minimum of 3 times and then repeat with the other leg. Do more if you sense that your body needs it.

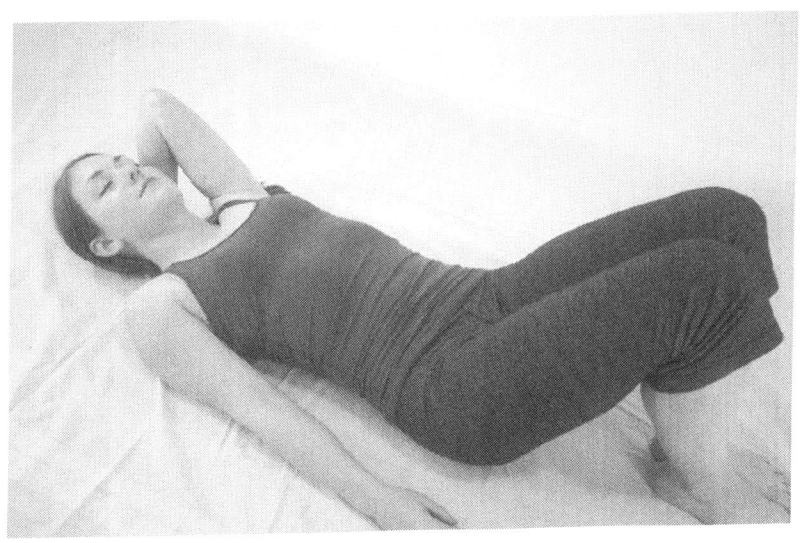

Prepare

Begin by lying flat on your back with your knees bent. Place your left hand behind your head with the palm up. Your right arm should remain by your side and your eyes should be closed.

Move Slowly

Inhale through your nose as you gently and slowly lift your left elbow towards your face. Take note of any sensations that you feel.

Release Slowly

Slowly exhale through your mouth as you lower your left elbow back to the ground.

Relax

Slowly inhale through your nose and exhale through your mouth. Focus your mind on whatever tension your feel and command those muscles to relax.

Repeat

Do this movement for a minimum of 3 times and then repeat with your right arm. Do more if you sense that your body needs it.

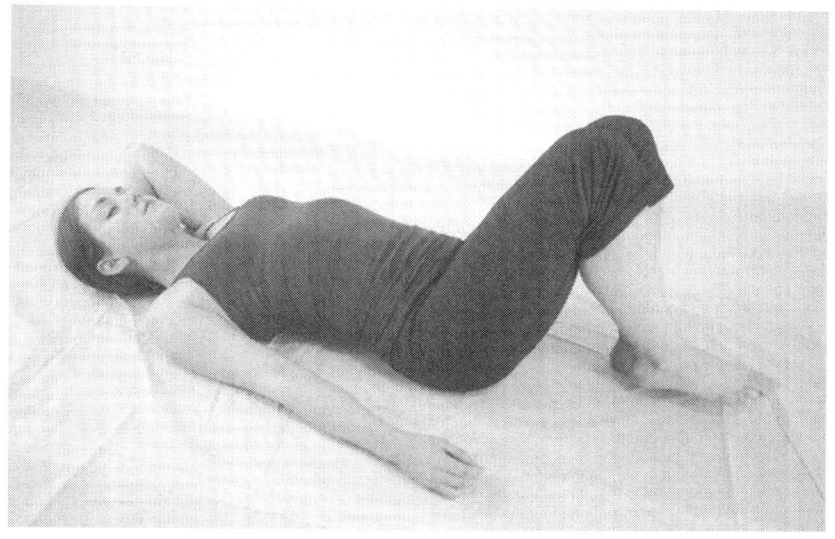

Prepare

Begin by lying flat on your back with your knees bent. Place your left hand behind your head with your palm up. Your right arm should remain by your side and your eyes should be closed.

Move Slowly

Inhale through your nose as you gently and slowly lift your left elbow towards your face. As you do so simultaneously and gently press your tailbone into the ground while you lift your right foot slightly off the ground.

Release Slowly

Slowly exhale through your mouth as you lower your left elbow and right foot back to the ground.

Relax

Slowly inhale through your nose and exhale through your mouth. Focus your mind on whatever tension your feel and command those muscles to relax.

Repeat

Do this movement for a minimum of 3 times and then repeat with your right arm and left leg. Do more if you sense that your body needs it.

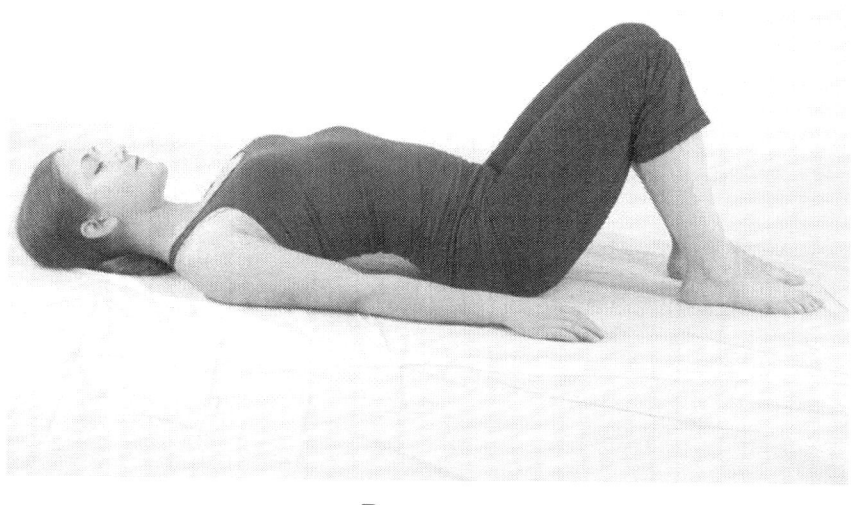

Prepare

You will now finish off with the first somatic movement you learned. Once again begin by lying flat on your back with your knees bent. As a variation though try starting with your feet closer together or further apart and see how this feels. Keep your eyes closed at all times.

Move Slowly

Inhale through your nose as you gently press your tailbone downwards. This will cause your lower back to arch up. Move slowly and focus on the sensations this movement causes within your body.

Release Slowly

Slowly exhale through your mouth as you gently thrust your pelvis slightly upward, which will flatten the arch in your back. Again focus on how your muscles feel as you do this. Take special note of any that seem to feel extra tense.

Relax

Slowly inhale through your nose and exhale through your mouth. As you do so focus your mind on the sensations you have just felt. If you felt any tension in your body focus your mind on relaxing those muscles.

Repeat

Do this movement for a minimum of 5 times. Do more if you sense that your body needs it.

Somatic Cat Stretch

As I've mentioned and you have likely observed all cats, both big and small, do what is commonly called a "Cat stretch" first thing in the morning. As you now know though they are not stretching as we know it, they are actually contracting and releasing their muscles. What follows is a somatic movement sequence that can be considered as the human equivalent of the cat stretch. It is a more advanced routine than either somatic sequence A and B, but it is also more thorough. If you feel you are getting great results from simply doing somatic sequences A or B there is nothing wrong with sticking with them. If, however, you want to try something more advanced and see how you feel give this human cat stretch a try. I think you will find it extremely beneficial.

Holistic Movement #1 – Human Cat Stretch

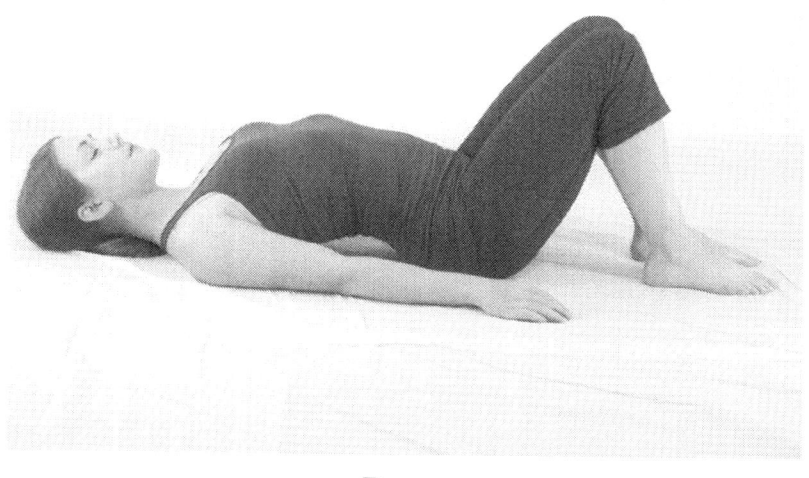

Prepare

Begin by lying flat on your back with your knees bent and your eyes closed.

Move Slowly

Inhale through your nose as you gently press your tailbone downwards. This will cause your lower back to arch up. Move slowly and focus on the sensations this movement causes within your body.

Release Slowly

Slowly exhale through your mouth as you gently thrust your pelvis slightly upward, which will flatten the arch in your back. Again focus on how your muscles feel as you do this. Take special note of any that seem to feel extra tense.

47

Relax

Slowly inhale through your nose and exhale through your mouth. As you do so focus your mind on the sensations you have just felt. If you felt any tension in your body focus your mind on relaxing those muscles.

Repeat

Do this movement for a minimum of 5 times. Do more if you sense that your body needs it.

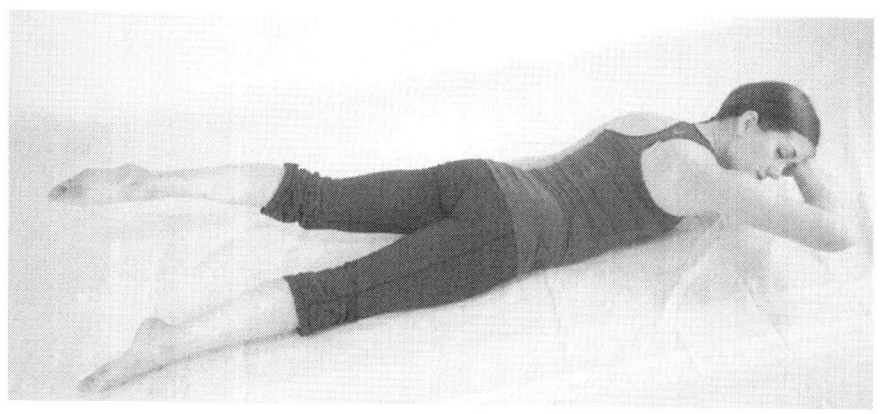

Prepare

Begin by lying flat on your stomach. Turn your head to the right and place your right hand under your left cheek. Your left arm should remain resting beside your body. Make sure that you close your eyes and keep them closed.

Move Slowly

Inhale through your nose as you slowly and gently lift your left leg a few inches off the floor along with your head, hand and elbow. You should feel no strain when doing this.

Release Slowly

Slowly exhale through your mouth as you lower your leg back to the ground.

Relax

Slowly inhale through your nose and exhale through your mouth. As you do so focus your mind on the sensations you have just felt. Did you feel any tension in your spine or shoulder? Focus your mind on relaxing those muscles or any area of your body where you felt tension.

Repeat

Do this movement for a minimum of 3 times. Then repeat this movement by reversing it (turning your head to the left and lifting your right leg).

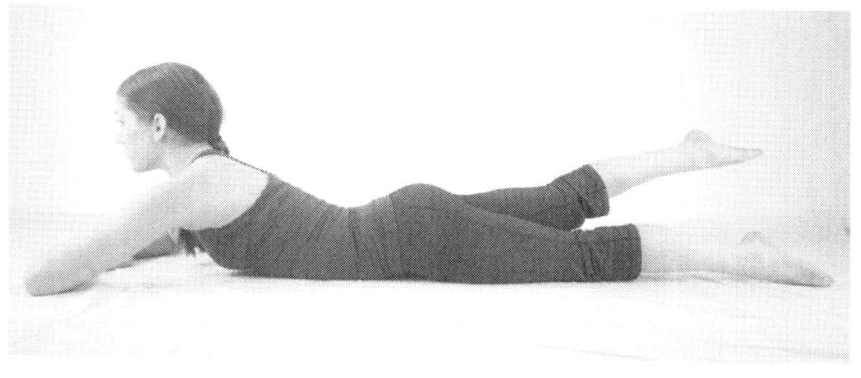

Prepare

Begin by lying flat on your stomach with your left hand over your right hand. Place the center of your forehead on the back of your hands and close your eyes.

Move Slowly

Inhale through your nose as you slowly and gently lift your right leg and head off the ground. Only move within your comfort zone. Focus on how your body feels.

Release Slowly

Slowly exhale through your mouth as you lower your leg and head to the ground.

Relax

Slowly inhale through your nose and exhale through your mouth as you relax your body. Breathe out any tension that you feel.

Repeat

Do this movement for a minimum of 3 times. When you are finished reverse the process by lifting your left leg and head 3 times in the same manner.

Holistic Movement #4 – Human Cat Stretch

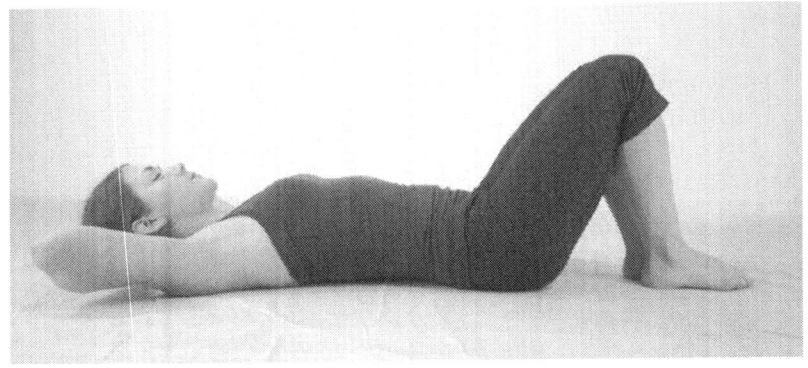

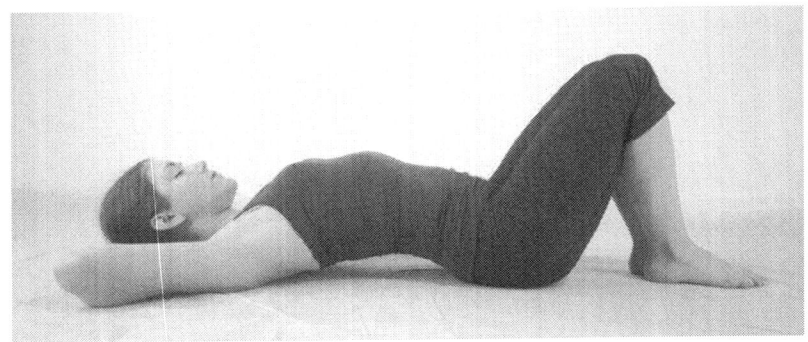

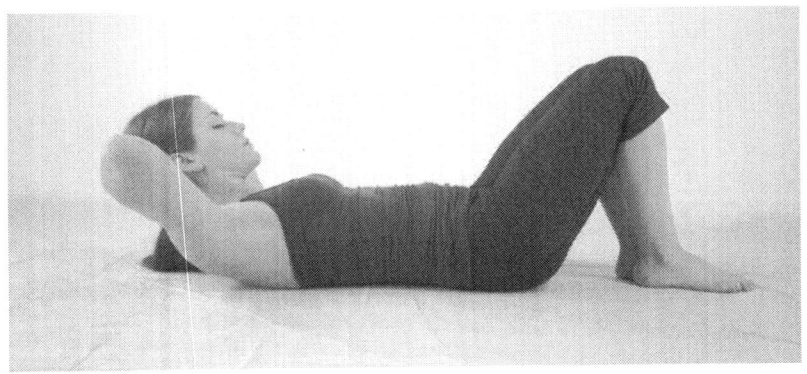

Holistic Movement #4 – Human Cat Stretch

Prepare

Begin on your back with your knees bent and your hands behind your head with your eyes closed.

Move Slowly

Inhale through your nose as you press your tailbone down into the floor. This will cause your back to arch. Do this slowly and gently.

Release Slowly

Slowly exhale through your mouth as you raise your pelvis and flatten your lower back to the ground while simultaneously lifting your head.

Relax

Slowly inhale through your nose and exhale through your mouth as you relax your body. Take note of any tension you feel and concentrate on relaxing those areas.

Repeat

Do this movement for a minimum of 5 times. You can do more if it feels good to you.

Holistic Movement #5 – Human Cat Stretch

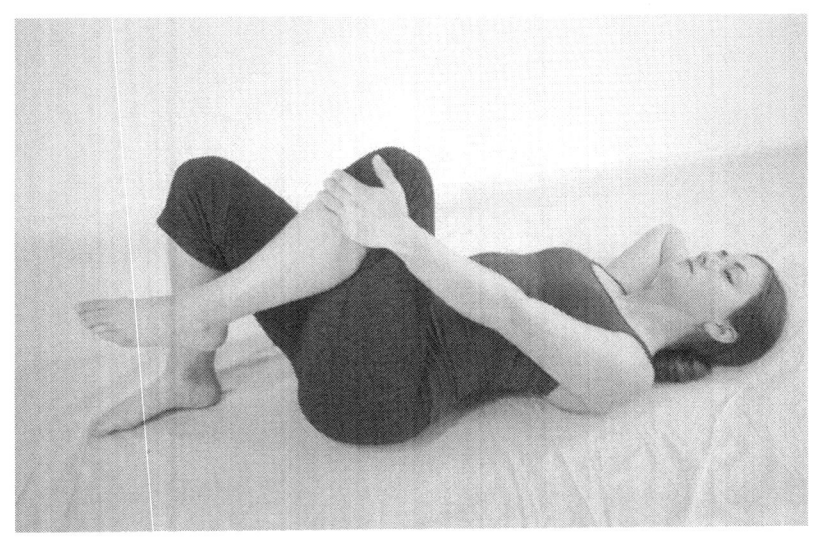

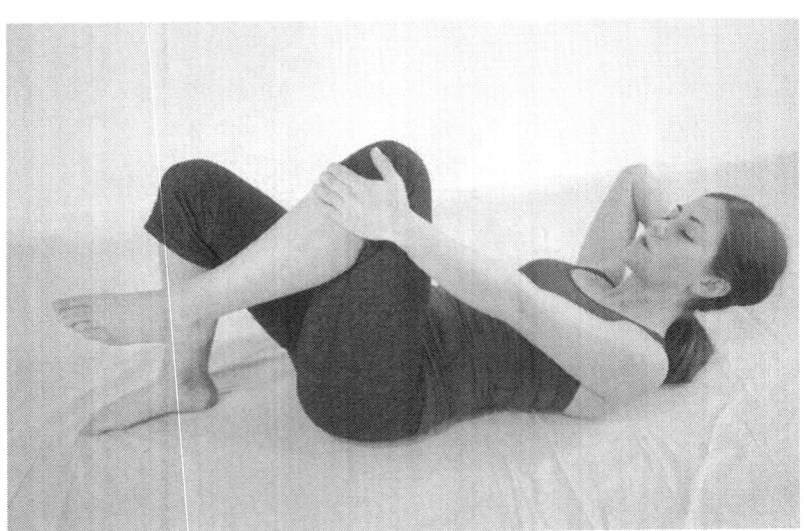

Holistic Movement #5 – Human Cat Stretch

Prepare

Begin on your back with your knees bent and your right hand behind your head. At the same time lift your left knee so that you can hold it with your left hand. Close your eyes.

Move Slowly

Inhale through your nose as you press your tailbone down into the floor, arching your lower back. Move slowly and gently. Really focus on how your back muscles feel.

Release Slowly

Slowly exhale through your mouth as you raise your pelvis and flatten your lower back to the ground while at the same time move your right elbow towards your left knee. It is not necessary to touch your elbow to your knee. Only move as far as it is comfortable, even if that is only an inch or two.

Relax

Slowly inhale through your nose and exhale through your mouth as you relax your body. However keep your hands on your head and knee as you relax. Focus your mind on relaxing your muscles.

Repeat

Do this movement for a minimum of 5 times. You can do more if it feels good to you. When you are finished repeat the movement with your left hand behind your head and your right hand on your right knee.

Holistic Movement #6 – Human Cat Stretch

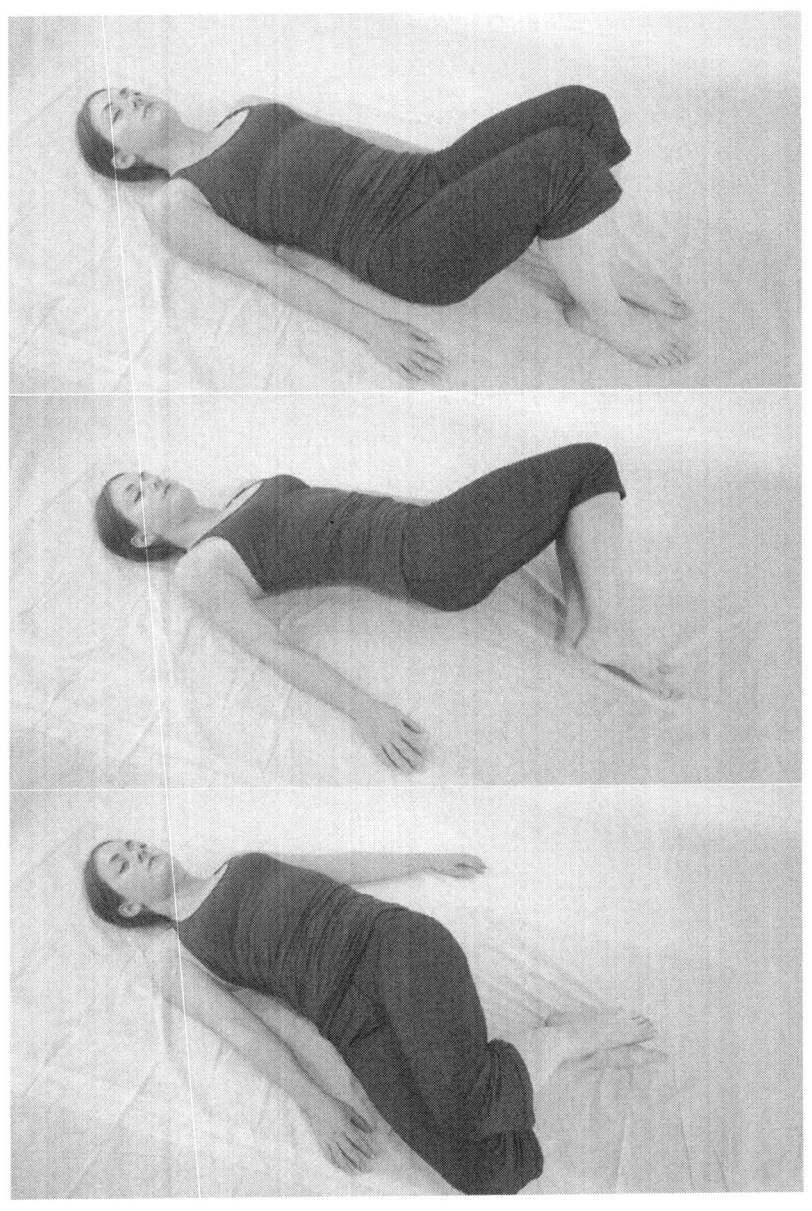

Holistic Movement #6 – Human Cat Stretch

Prepare

Begin on your back with both of your knees comfortably bent. This is the neutral position. Close your eyes.

Move Slowly

Inhale through your nose as you slowly drop both of your knees to the left.

Release Slowly

Exhale through your mouth as you return your knees to the neutral position.

Relax

Slowly inhale through your nose and exhale through your mouth as you focus your mind on relaxing your muscles.

Repeat

Repeat this movement but this time allow your knees to drop to the right. This constitutes one set. Repeat this movement for another four sets.

Holistic Movement #7 – Human Cat Stretch

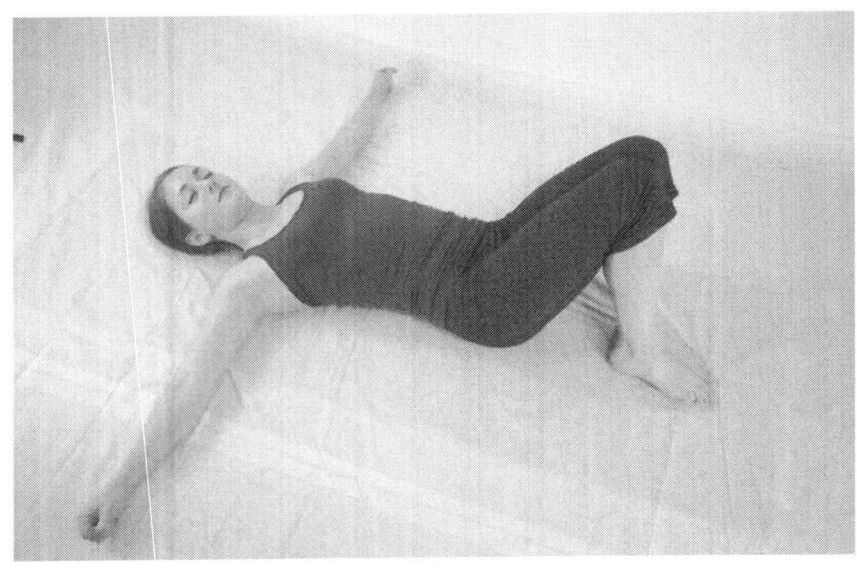

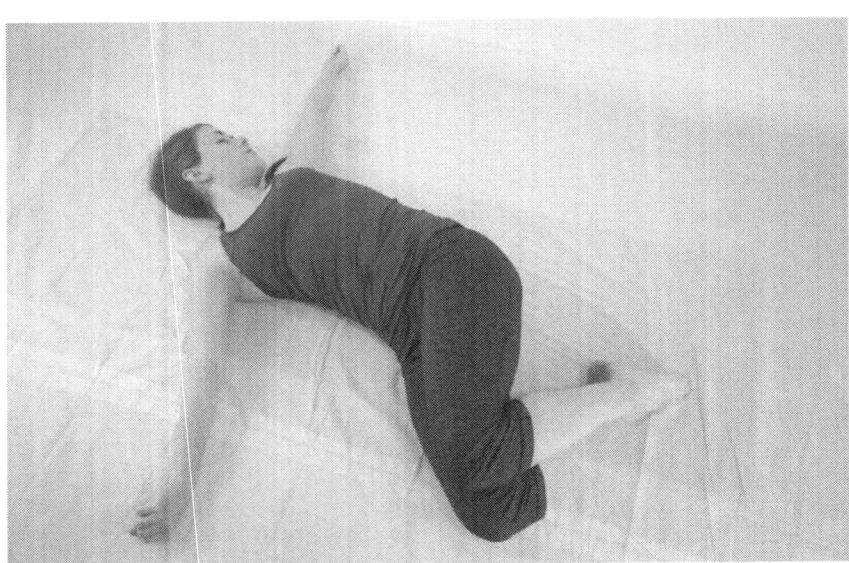

Holistic Movement #7 – Human Cat Stretch

Prepare

Begin on your back with your knees bent and both of your arms stretched out perpendicular to your sides. Close your eyes. This is the neutral position.

Move Slowly

Inhale through your nose as you simultaneously do the following:

- Roll your left arm upward and your right hand downwards. Do not slide your arms. This will not be a large movement as you can only rotate your arms so far. This should slightly press your left shoulder down while raising your right shoulder.
- Let your two legs drop down to the right.
- Roll your head to the left.

Release Slowly

Slowly exhale through your mouth as you return your body to the neutral position. Do this slowly, almost lazily. Think of how a cat stretches in the morning.

Relax

Slowly inhale through your nose and exhale through your mouth as you relax your body. Take note of how your muscles feel and allow them to relax.

Repeat

Now repeat this movement moving in reverse (rolling your left arm downwards, letting your legs drop to the left, etc.). This counts as one repetition. Do a minimum of six of these or more if you feel your body needs it.

FAQ

I can see how these somatic movements could be really beneficial for flexibility and pain management, but can anyone really do them?

These movements can literally benefit everyone and can be done by anybody. It doesn't matter whether you're an athlete in your twenties or a senior citizen. So long as you perform these movements slowly and stay well within your comfort zone you will be fine. It's all about rebooting your brain and anyone can do it.

I want to do these somatic movements but I'm so stiff I can't even lie flat on the ground currently. What should I do?

If your muscles are so tight that you can't even get into the most basic positions feel free to use pillows to make it comfortable for you. For example if you cannot even lie flat on the ground put some firm pillows underneath your legs or back so that you are lying comfortably without strain. From there just do the movements to the best of your ability. With time your muscles will start to relax and you should be able to lie on the floor normally.

My body has really broken down and I can barely move. What can I do?

People find this hard to believe, but you can benefit from these movements without moving at all. All you need to do is imagine that you are doing them and you'll still get benefits. You do need to concentrate with laser like focus, but it does work. The reason for this is that you are training your mind with somatic movements, not your muscles. If your mind thinks it is doing the movements you will gain the benefits. Performing the movements is really just a way to focus your mind.

There was a famous experiment done that demonstrates this principle. A group of people were divided into three groups and told to shoot basketball free throws. One of the groups then spent some time everyday for a few weeks practicing free throws. When they were tested again they showed remarkable improvement. The second group didn't practice at all (they were the control group) and not surprisingly demonstrated no improvement. The third group simply spent some time everyday visualizing improving their foul shots. When they were tested again, they showed almost the same improvement as the first group who had actually practiced. What this dramatically shows is that it is the mind that controls the muscles. When you practice anything physical you are really training your mind. This is why you can get benefits from simply visualizing doing these movements if you can't do them physically. Always remember that somatic movements are a method for training and rebooting your mind, not your muscles.

I've been doing these movements but my muscles seem to be getting tighter, not looser. What am I doing wrong?

Most likely you are going to fast and trying to hard. If you do not perform these movements slowly with focused intent you run the risk of using your subcortical brain as opposed to your cortical. If you don't seem to be improving turning it down a gear and going slower is always a good idea.

I've read what you've written but I'm still confused about this cortical and subcortical brain stuff. Can you explain it to me again?

Here's another way to look at it. When you are first learning a new skill you are using your cortical brain. Think back when you learned to drive, for example. At first you're thinking about everything as you learn this new skill. As you get better at it though it almost becomes automatic, the intense thought process fades into the background. You no longer need to think about every little thing when you drive to the store, it's almost automatic. At this point you are using your subcortical brain. This is why it is critical that when you are trying to reset the instructions in your subcortical brain that you move slowly and really think about the muscles that you are using. When you are thinking about and feeling the muscles work you are using your cortical brain. With time this will reprogram your subcortical brain and rejuvenate you. When you go fast, however, you are using your subcortical brain and nothing will change. I know I sound like a broken record but going slowly with conscious intention is the key to the kingdom.

When I perform these movements my mind tends to wander. Is there anything I can do about this?

This is normal and the last thing you want to do is to get stressed out over it as this would be extremely counter-productive. Just keep

65

working on it and your mental focus can't help but improve. Just like it takes time to build the stamina to run a marathon it takes time to build your mental focus. Be patient, work at it and it will come.

I often feel a little sleepy after completing some of these somatic movements. Is this normal?

When you are performing somatic movements properly your brain will be releasing chemicals to relax your muscles that can often lead to a feeling of sleepiness. This is completely normal and the feeling will pass as you get up and get on with your day.

How many repetitions should I do?

For all of the movements I suggest a minimum number to perform. However, as your body begins to reset itself you may find that you can do less. On the other hand if you've experienced some kind of trauma you may find that more repetitions are beneficial on a particular day. Ultimately it's all up to you and how your body feels. Listen to your body and you'll be fine.

This book is great but I'm looking to take it to the next level. Are you planning on putting out a more advanced book?

Not at this time. However, if you are looking to try different kinds of somatic movements I recommend getting "Somatics" by Thomas Hanna. Hanna is really a pioneer is this kind of sports medicine therapy and his book contains many more somatic movements that you may wish to try later on. My only criticism of the book is that it can be slightly confusing to read and, in my opinion, he doesn't stress the necessity of moving slowly enough. Nonetheless it is an excellent book and well worth your time.

About the Author

Anthony Anholt has been interested and involved in athletics and fitness for his entire life. His specialty is "gymless" workouts, or exercise systems that do not require any kind of special equipment. He is also interested in enhancing performance in all sports, but particularly basketball. This is his seventh book.

About the Model

Dana Sorensen is a Vancouver based fitness instructor, performer and dancer. She can be contacted for modeling work here: http://www.modelmayhem.com/1709968

One Last Thing

You've now reached the end of the book and I hope it has helped you to restore your body to a more youthful and pain free state. If you did find it useful I would very much appreciate it if you could take 5 minutes and write a short review for it on Amazon or wherever you purchased it. Even a couple of sentences would be immensely helpful to me. Regardless I want to thank-you once again for purchasing my book and I wish you all the best in the future.

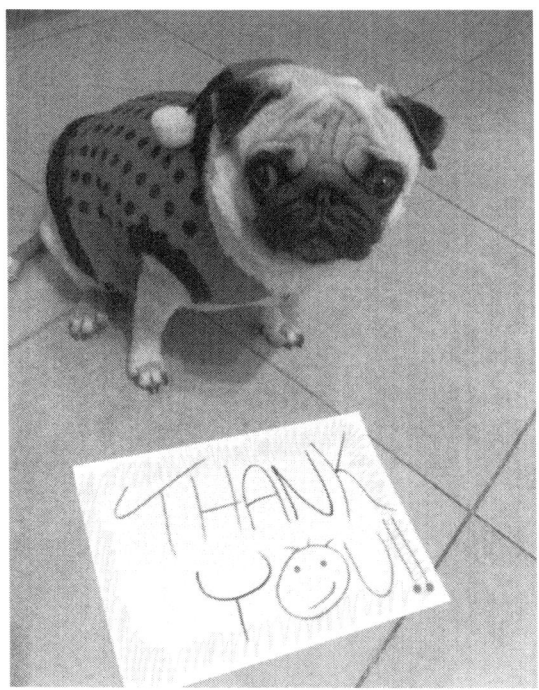

39019848R10041

Made in the USA
San Bernardino, CA
17 September 2016